WELCOME TO CAMP I
LET'S GET BETTER

GETTING THE MOST OUT OF TREATMENT

VOLUME I

HAMILTON PEIRSOL, PSY. D.
2ND EDITION ©2019
SAVANNAH, GEORGIA

AMAZON PRESS

INTRODUCTION

Welcome to Camp I: Let's Get Better provides supportive, light-hearted "tips" on successfully completing an intensive psychotherapeutic treatment program such as residential treatment, a PHP or day-treatment, an IOP, or even outpatient treatment, a.k.a. "Camp!" This book is essentially a thrifty little endurance guide for Camp. The suggestions are literal and specific to treatment on the one hand, as well as reflective and figurative to life in general on the other hand. *Welcome to Camp* assists in taking the sting out of the idea of going to Camp in the first place. It instills and empowers a curiosity and hope rather than the fear and dismay typically found at Camp; and, for an Aristotelian final cause, it provides some objectivity and direction to guide and ease the natural tensions surrounding what otherwise are very serious and arduous life lessons to be learned at Camp along the way.

I discovered as a counselor many patients get lost in all the ends and outs of a treatment program. There is a lot of mystery around how all of it works and as a result, many end up not getting all they might need from the experience. First and foremost, patients are generally numb, in somewhat of a shock, and feeling mostly displaced when they first come into a treatment setting. They might not be at all sure of themselves; and. whatever decisions they are making at first are generally deferred to the staff. As a result, they can easily get lost in all the drama, taking them several days if not weeks to get their barring. In the end, they may end up getting just enough of what they need to land on their feet, but not all of what they could have gained to help them stay on their feet when they get out.

Let's Get Better: Welcome to Camp is written for those who may be experiencing their first treatment setting and for those who might have been to Camp multiple times. Ultimately, *Welcome to Camp* is for anyone who wants to be successful in their treatment experience so they can get what they need once and for all and avoid the need for additional treatment stays.

This book is an effort to provide insight about the treatment experience almost *in vivo* so you can either be prepared before something happens or while it is happening at Camp. It attempts to prepare you as quickly as possible, sometimes on the spot, for making the most of your treatment involvement. It intends to take you as close to the heart of the matter while you are actually there to assist you in processing your understanding more effectively.

For example, there is the phenomena "counter-transference" in the field of psychology. All therapists are human, but sometimes they get lost in their own stuff while helping others. As a result, they end up letting their own issues interfere with what the patient is trying to resolve. Being able to minimize the impact of this, if it does arise while at Camp, is critical and might make the difference in whether or not the treatment experience is a good one or not for you.

It's rough enough showing up for treatment much less trying to find your way through it. In this book *Welcome to Camp*, I might not be able to help you pick up specifically on your own therapist's "counter-transference" issues, if you will, but we might be able to minimize the impact of it if we have to simply by knowing to ask certain questions of our therapist beforehand.

Ideally of course, it's better if you are coming on your own volition to Camp but if you aren't then these tips might be even more enlightening and provide you with certain short cuts to managing your treatment experience while there. The idea is "Well, if you have to go then you might as well get the most out of it!" In other words, there are things you can do to get the most out of Camp and in the end not regret it at all.

For example, first and foremost, there are people counting on you even if they are counting on you to just make sure you take better care of yourself. Hence, life is not all about just you anymore even though Camp's primary focus is on you. The intention is ultimately help you connect primarily with yourself so you can better connect in turn with others. Second, you can do it! Many have been successful before you and immeasurably gained from their Camp experience. Third, if you are concerned about what it may cost you now, I can assure you it will cost you more later. Fourth, whatever condition or situation you may be facing, you were not meant to deal with it alone. Now might be the time to share the burden. Fifth, there is help out there and this might be the first step in a better direction. Everybody can change so now is as good a time as any. Hence, those are just tidbits of what's more to come in *Welcome to Camp*.

Now, as a caveat, some people like to just show up and let what happens happen. That's okay, too. Not all of these tips may fit you in other words. As you go through the tips, let the ones that speak to you help you along the way. Those that don't fit initially, come back to them later as you go through Camp. Sometimes certain tips make more sense the further along you go within your Camp experience.

Since it has been said that wisdom is the principle thing and that we should get as much of it as we can, we are also reminded that with all that getting we need to get understanding. As a result, *Welcome to Camp* is here to provide you with enough understanding about certain aspects of treatment so you can be wise in your efforts to make the most of Camp.

This book is devoted to all of those that are searching to find the answers to make their life work more fluidly, more effectively, so it will run more smoothly without so much effort. It is an applause to all those who have endured the process and lived to talk about it. It is also for those who long to be whole, to find their way and make a mark for themselves in this world. It is for the broken-hearted who struggle with finding more meaning to their loss and for the forlorn who wonder if all the effort of getting well is really worth it. It is for the victorious who have been there and done that, capable of looking back now with pride on the achievement of recovery itself.

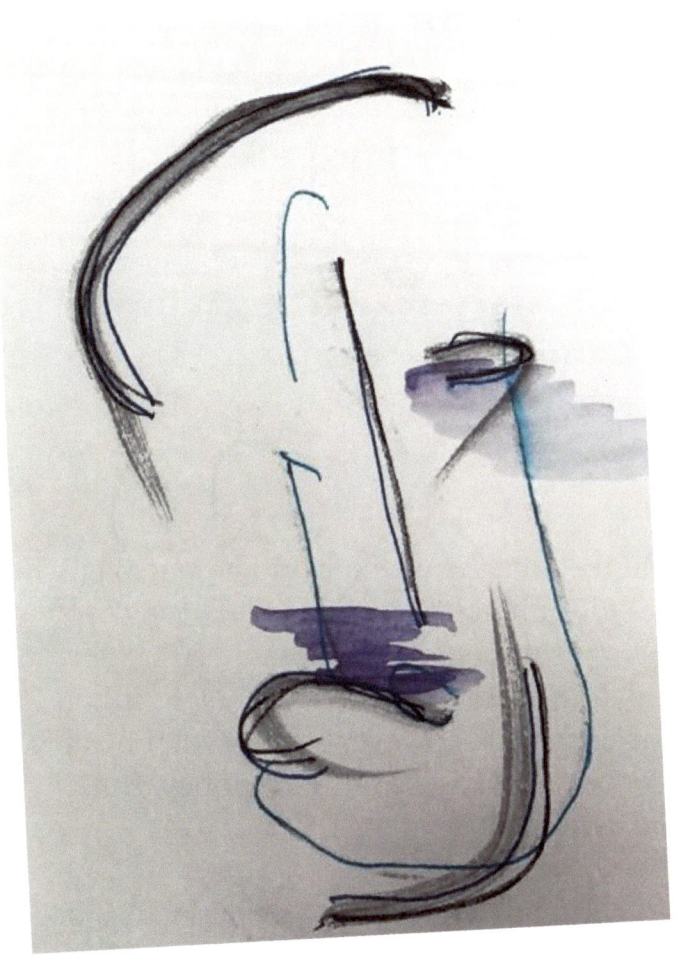

Determined. Better Outcomes

Retitled watercolor on paper canvas with sketch tones
©2019 DR. PEIRSOL

TIPS

1. For starters, just making it to Camp is a fete unto itself. Do not spoil it by worrying about how you look.

It might feel like the whole world is watching when you get to Camp but do not sweat it - as if you are not feeling self-conscious enough as it is already. You might even try to get there at night if you feel too self-conscious however you may not be able to pull this one off because of Camp policy. But, if you can, it is worth a try.

Here is the tendency- to want to not look as bad as you may feel. The good news is feeling bad is good when you go to Camp. It is counterintuitive. The worse you feel, the better off you will be at Camp to start.

2. From the start, do not expect to know all the ins-and-outs of Camp. Just be glad you made it even though you might equally hate the fact you are there in the first place.

Everything that has led to this moment is significant and most likely very overwhelming if you were to try to ever dissect if fully. So, do not even try. You realistically cannot sort it out right now. Besides, the first 24 to 48-hours are the toughest anyway at Camp. Instead, take the position you are cruising into Camp with a view that this experience is simply a new chapter in your life. Do this rather than be consumed by all the baggage you are feeling every which way. It is too much. You see, we can focus on all the problems we are feeling if we want to; or, we can paint the picture Camp is a new lease on life. Perspective at this point is everything. It helps and the sooner you can get one the better off you will be.

3. First and foremost, be kind to the charge nurse. They handle the meds.

Now this sounds pretty simple and of course you are probably a very considerate person at that; but, the charge nurse may be the primary person available to get you the medical attention you may need. They are very, very important. They communicate primarily with the attending physicians and are basically the hub for the staff in the delivery of the clinical protocol. Some nurses can be warm and fuzzy but if they are busy, they might be cold and calculated- saying all the right things but not really able to fully be there for you. The issue is that the nurse(s) sometimes get really busy and they are like anybody else- they can tend to cater to those they prefer over and above those they do not per se, especially when it is crunch time on their shift. Believe me, there are plenty of Campers they definitely might not favor so do not be one of them because some charge nurses can be quite particular. This does not mean be a brown nose toward them. They catch onto that real fast and think you are manipulative. I am just telling you they can be a life-line when you need them so make sure you start this relationship out right.

4. Make sure you have the "intake" counselors, or the charge nurses introduce you to your primary physician ASAP. Asking for more and getting less is better than asking for less and not getting enough.

The "good-doctor" is a key-master and the gate-keeper. Ask if you can meet with them regularly. That is right. Be bold. Constant check-ups are a good thing at Camp. The sooner you get off on a good clinical direction the better. Remember, you are not there for long even though at the start it might feel like forever. Realistically, the doctor might not be able to meet with you as often as you would like but at least he or she knows you mean business.

To receive the best care available, clinicians need time with you to diagnose properly. The more time they have the better the diagnosis. You need as much exposure as the doctor needs exposure to you. Why? Well, there is a puzzle to put together and the puzzle is you. You have to make sure they have all the pieces and that can take time.

5. Early on, ask nicely to meet the clinical director, too. They oversee all the professional help you will be getting. Now that you are getting started, it is nice to know who has your back.

You simply want to make sure the clinical director knows who you are in case something does not run smoothly during Camp. The clinical director might be the lead clinician for example. Just keep in mind there are a lot of idiosyncrasies going on behind the scenes at Camp. Everybody has issues and some more than others- therapists included! The clinical director is director because they generally function above the fray (not all but most) and they monitor the barometer of Camp: the good, the bad, the indifferent, and ultimately the ugly.

If possible, it is a good idea to know who is in charge from the get-go. Do not be too pushy though because it will come off as being "controlling." It is kind of an unspoken mantra at Camp: any Camper asking too many questions or one who has an answer for most of the questions is kind of offensive to the staff- it is a turn off for all sorts of reasons, some clinical and some not, all of which you need not bother with right now. The key here is to just be causal about this or your attempt could set you back and you do not want that. All you are wanting to do is make sure you are known (in a positive light of course) especially for the fact you are committed to the process, that you respect the Director's authority; and, most importantly, you both understand at the outset you will look to them for guidance if need be in a pinch.

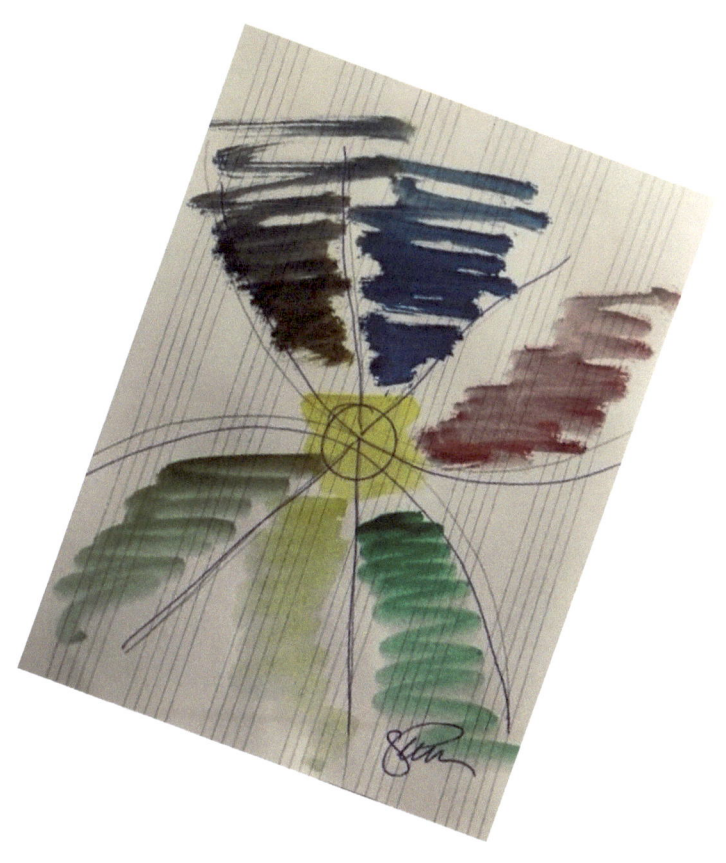

6. It may take a few days at some Campsites, but when you first meet your "assigned" therapist, be sure to ask them a bunch of questions, too. Getting help is a two-way street.

If your therapist gets defensive or noticeably evasive when asking them questions, it might be time to have some lunch with the clinical director. This one is really important. In some Camps you really do not have the luxury of changing your therapist if the one you get does not rub you the right way. But if you have the option then the idea is to have as good a fit as possible. And, if you cannot change therapists, then you at least know what you are dealing with from the start by asking a few simple questions.

Remember, clinicians have issues, too. They are human just like you. And, many times, those who are counselors have had their share of issues lead them to their being really good counselors. It is important though their issues not interfere with what you need. So, in that first meeting, you want to filter through any potential issues that may arise between the two of you.

Some good questions might be "How did you get into the field? How long have you been in the field? Given what issues I'm dealing with, do you feel these issues would be disruptive for you in any way?" If you are not really comfortable with some of their responses or how they respond, then the idea is to talk about it up front. Get everything out on the table. If after talking about it, and it still does not pan out, amicably ask for an alternate consideration or a chance to talk to the Clinical Director. Believe me, it is worth the effort because you invariably have to deal with your therapist most every day while at Camp so why not get the one that best fits you if you can.

If after all that, and nothing has changed, it will still be okay because your therapist and you can work it out over time and that might be some of the work you need to do anyway as part of the reason you are at Camp in the first place. You will soon discover everything starts to have a purpose and a reason for being the way it is as you go along, therapists included.

7. After meeting your therapist and the clinical director, ask nicely when you can talk to the aftercare counselor as well. They help organize your discharge plan. Now that you are in, it is nice to know who is going to be helping you get out.

Do not do this immediately but certainly within the first two-weeks after you have met your therapist. Many times, your therapist will actually function as the discharge counselor in some settings, so be sure to talk "aftercare" with them first regardless. Not going through the right channels or asking some questions too soon might suggest to the staff you are not committed to the process or you are controlling treatment and that is not a good start.

Remember, this treatment is for you, so it needs to be a comprehensive approach, from soup to nuts, from beginning to end, and aftercare is just as critical as the beginning care. Pace yourself on the one hand but equally know where you are headed while at Camp when you can. The key here is to get the discharge preparations started because the most important part of treatment for some is going to be the aftercare anyway. Aftercare is where you have to put it all together when you get out. Besides, therapists start treatment upon admission with a discharge plan in mind so why shouldn't you?

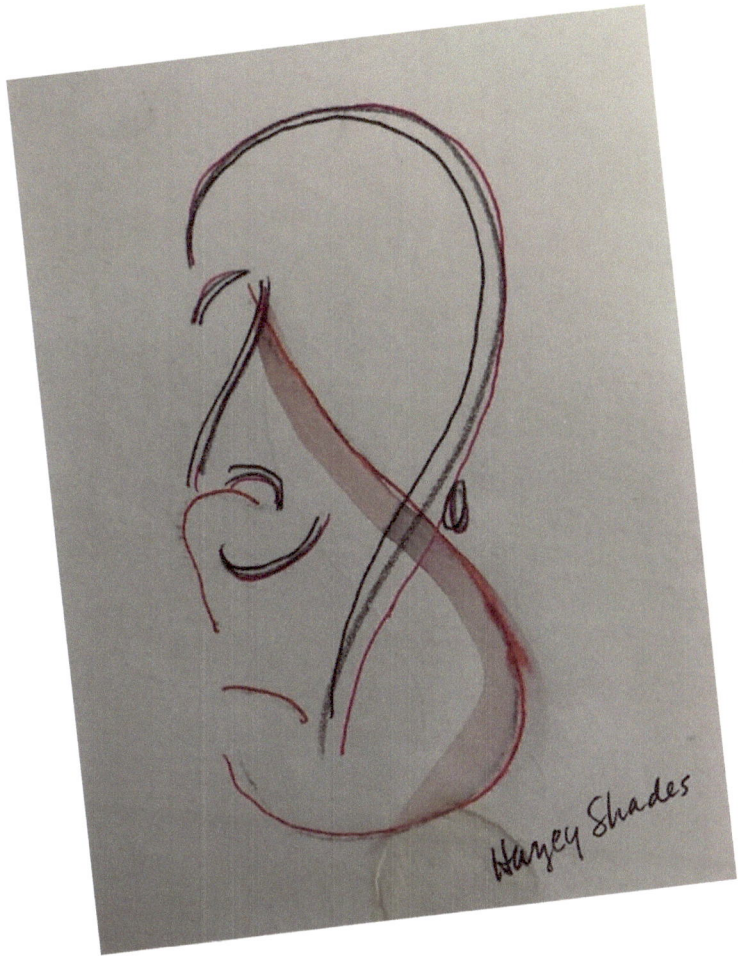

8. Look for those folks who seem to be the most laid back. Hang out with them at first if you can. They might already have an edge on getting settled in. At Camp, "easy going" is a good thing at the "get-go."

Those who are little more relaxed in treatment might be the more seasoned Campers who have been there a while. If they are in a "good place," or at least appear to be, then they must have learned a thing or two about how to do it. There is no use reinventing the wheel if you do not have to. Ask them for any suggestions that might help you get better quicker. The more ropes you can learn the better. They might give you some hard-earned advice you would not know otherwise. Besides, it is for a lack of knowledge we hurt ourselves so remember it never hurts to ask.

9. Start gravitating toward those who laugh a lot, especially those who tell great jokes. They will help you feel better adjusted even if it is just a brief illusion.

I am serious about this one. Without fail, whenever you hang around the funny Campers you definitely feel better. In fact, while at Camp you might not remember laughing so hard especially if you make these kinds of connections. Go out of your way to run into some funny Campers because they can make all the difference. If anything, they are just enjoyable to be with. Take the time to get to know them and hang out with them as often as you can. Every little bit helps.

10. It is important to try to start slow, be clear, and ease your way into sharing your feelings during those first couple days. You want people to get you as you get going.

People who get it get what is real so be as real as you can. If anything, just say you are angry you ended up having to come to Camp; that you did not know what you needed to know to stay out of Camp! It will be strange at first because you really do not know what to say at times; and yet, you are expected to jump right in and start sharing, spilling your guts.

It is okay to not ever really be sure what to say when but at least try. The good news is, it all comes out in the wash eventually. The reason to take it slowly at first is so you can gather your thoughts if you can. If you can't seem to collect them, then just let them rip. The idea here, if you can, make sure you cultivate as much support as possible up front; that people understand you as best they can as soon as they can. This helps ensure solid support for you from the "get-go."

11. Take a warm shower as often as you can. Why? It just feels good.

Why put this one in here you might ask. Well, the bottom line is you are away from the comforts of home and we tend to do better when we can re-create what is familiar. So, why not get a head start just in feeling better? Everybody likes a warm shower. It is easy. No restrictions. All you have to do is jump in. Besides, it is a diversion and you can daydream all you want when you are in there. Oh, go ahead, take one. It works!

12. Sign up early to talk on the phone. Depending on your Campsite, there are only a few phones and those who talk a lot tend to be pretty controlling.

Just trying to get on the phone is not always fun. Nothing worse than longing to talk to someone you care about, away from all the chaos of Camp, and having to wait in line for somebody else to get off the darn phone. Not everybody sticks to the time limits set for the phones either. You only have so much time before you have got to be somewhere else; so, sign up fast, get in line early, and enjoy a relaxed non-rushed call with someone you want to talk to. It could make all the difference.

13. When you have that first phone call with a loved one, it is okay to say you will need more than "sympathy" cards sent to you. Who knows, you might get that Tommy Bahamas sweat shirt you have always wanted.

Little consolations here and there go a long way; but, after a "very short" while, you will need more than cards. Cards and all that are very meaningful from the very beginning. It is nice to read everyone's well-wishing thoughts for you and their warm gestures of "Hurry home!" But, after a while, you need something more tangible. One mom sent a colorful little wooden fish to remind her daughter of the ocean. Don't knock it. It worked! It was the next best thing to being there.

14. Do not call friends and family and do all the talking either. Have them fill you in on their lives, too. Listening to others sometimes helps you see another world while you feel lost in your own.

You will find that phone calls are a nice escape. And, believe me, you need as many escapes as you can get while you are at Camp. To take it a step further, it is really important to hear stories of what is happening at home if not for any other reason than to imagine what it would be like if you were there.

15. Early on, get outside and get some fresh air. Once those wheels start spinning, it is really easy to get all spun out.

One woman got so spun out at Camp she started pulling out her own hair! The lesson here is 1) take it easy 2) take small breaks, and 3) try to take it all in but remember it is important to let some of it go.

We are human and feeling broken is a part of the journey. It is not the exception either at this point. It is the rule. And, it is okay to start getting used to how fragile you might be feeling right now.

16. Observe those who are the loudest in the bunch. They generally have connections with those in charge.

Inevitably, there is always some Camper getting in trouble and getting the so-called pink slip. They are usually the loudest in the bunch. Too many pink slips though mean they have to go before the clinical team to determine whether or not they get to stay.

The people managing these troublesome Campers are the ones you want to meet; however, there are other ways to meet them! You have to figure, if they have that much power to throw someone out then they must have the power to help someone stay in. So, introduce yourself to these pink slip recipients and ask them who is in charge, who they have to meet and who you should be sure to meet. In other words, you want to meet as many members of the clinical team whenever possible. They can help you stay in good stead or get out of trouble; whichever need comes first.

17. In-group therapy, listen at first if you can rather than just jump right in. Listening sometimes can help to put your story in better perspective.

You are the newcomer and generally do not know dittlely-squat about what has been happening in the group long before you joined. Wait until you hear some of the other Campers' stories first if you can. You are welcome to jump right in though if you want; however, remember the idea of group is in large part about your ability to connect with the other members in the group. To make this work though, one usually has to work through any disconnections that might surface along the way. That is why you want to try to connect as well as you can up front so there are fewer issues to deal with later. Believe me; issues will come up anyway so you cannot avoid that. Just try to pace yourself is the key here. The less unnecessary problems you bring on yourself the better in other words.

18. When you are sitting at your first meal, and you have no clue of anyone around you, just wait and sit still, savor the bites as best you can until a socialite Camper type swings by. Be patient, they will come; and, when they do, just let them talk. Keep in mind, they are the connection you might need when Camp starts to get really tough.

There generally is someone at Camp who is the social butterfly. They usually take the lead in organizing the social aspects of Camp. Get to know them if you can because they are generally connected to those in charge politically, organizing and arranging activities that might impact you. It is always a good idea to afford yourself a good relationship here because you never know which of you might need a favor. Remember, even at Camp, it is good to be connected.

19. Also, after a while, depending on your Campsite, sit in different places with different people when you eat. It will help you feel less stuck.

I do not know what it is, but we are genuinely creatures of habit. We tend to gravitate toward what is familiar once it exists. The problem though is we are at Camp to change old habits and to get new ones. So, why not change your seating habits while you eat? Besides, this can break up some of the monotony. Depending upon the size of your Camp, you meet new people and get exposed to new ideas just from the conversations you might have with a stranger, who is in all actuality a sojourner with you along the way.

20. As you go along, stop worrying too much about how you keep looking. Things can get pretty ugly at Camp.

Good hygiene and all that is important so be sure to keep up with that but do not overdo it. The key is you are in a place to simply be who you are in whatever which way you are at any given time. Yes, you might want to look presentable of course but do not get caught up in it. Time is precious and you only have so much of it to address whatever in the world you need to. No need to waste it on unnecessary primping or worries about how you will look or appear to others. Remember, what you are doing is for you, so you feel better not just look better. Besides, the more genuine you are, even if at times it is pretty ugly, the more authentically beautiful it will become later anyway.

21. Do not forget, Camp is a twisted way of helping us "grow up." Sometimes we have to feel really bad before we can feel really good.

This one is painful, but it is clear: the further along we go in life the more grown up we have to become. How we feel and what we do can sometimes be two separate things. Know whatever you have that is emotionally charged, or otherwise in your life, has to be embraced and properly reintegrated. Always remember that whatever it is you may be dealing with, however bad it might be for you to feel, you are going to be okay because you are with other similarly struggling campers.

More importantly, you have a bunch of Campmates with you who have an equally vested interest in getting better, too. Remember, there is always strength in numbers. In fact, keep in mind that along the way you will probably feel worse first. Take heart, that just means you are on the verge of feeling better. The bigger the problem the greater the relief. Once you get to the other side of feeling bad, it is like "Wow, never thought it could be so good!"

22. If not already, you are eventually going to begin to feel really vulnerable at Camp. The key is to remember this is a great sign you are headed in the right direction.

The more vulnerable you are at first suggests the more real and genuine you can possibly become. The "real" you gets a chance to come out and be presented for just the way you are rather than the way you might have always felt or thought you needed to be. At first, you might think this vulnerability will push people away. It does just the opposite. When you are vulnerably real and genuine about who you are or how you feel, regardless of how bad it may be, people are generally drawn closer to you. Plus, the added benefit is you are normally more respected in the end because they finally are getting to know just how human-like you truly are. The more human the better.

23. Always be considerate of your Campmates. You can be firm but be considerate. A lot of them will probably be attending your "closing ceremony" when you spill your guts about how helpful everyone was, what you learned, and how much better you feel because of them.

You are writing your new story every day at Camp and others are reading the daily headlines on how you are doing. If you are doing the work day-in and day-out, those around you will get to know you for who you really are. Some will like you and some will not; but nobody will be able to take away your being yourself along the way. Most people can considerately acknowledge most anyone who can respectfully be honest with themselves and respectfully support others in the process.

24. Take a notebook and pen to class. You do not want to feel any more stupid than you already feel.

There are a bunch of psycho-educational groups being conducted usually at Camp. For most Campers, information overload is a generous way of putting it the further along you go. So, the fact is you usually will not be able to take it all in. Thus, a little note taking for later review is a good idea. Besides, it will certainly convey you are at least interested even though at times you most certainly will not be. There are certain saturation points and they vary from camper-to-camper. Face it, there may be too much on your mind or you could simply be feeling exhausted, etc.; nonetheless, some note taking will help you stay focused for the most part if you are not.

The idea is you do not want to miss a nugget of truth if you can help it; and, here is the kicker, sometimes those moments of "aha" truths can come when you least expect them. Something someone said or something someone did can make all the difference sometimes. Whatever it may be, the healing moments come at any time during Camp; and yes, even while taking notes!

25. At first, always get to your therapy sessions on time and not fashionably late; otherwise, you might get labeled as "avoidant, passive-aggressive, co-dependent, narcissistic," or something else, only to name a few. But hey, who knows, you might become a therapist someday and need to know all these terms anyway.

Nothing at Camp goes uninterpreted. Your gait is even evaluated so you have to know how you manage your time will be, too. Your therapist does not know you at all to start so they are very keen in reading you at first. They have to get their bearings on you and position themselves therapeutically to best serve you. In the end, in the final analysis, your therapist relationship is one with whom you get mirrored back what you might not be seeing in yourself. For that to happen, you and your therapist need some time to get to know each other. So, avoid unnecessary exchanges of information at first if you can, such as being late. Instead, protect the time you have with them so it can be less interrupted. You might begin to talk about the obvious with your therapist if you cannot figure out what is hidden underneath your feelings; and, if need be, that might include why you are late if in fact that happens. What is blatantly obvious can sometimes be the gateway to that which otherwise has been lost.

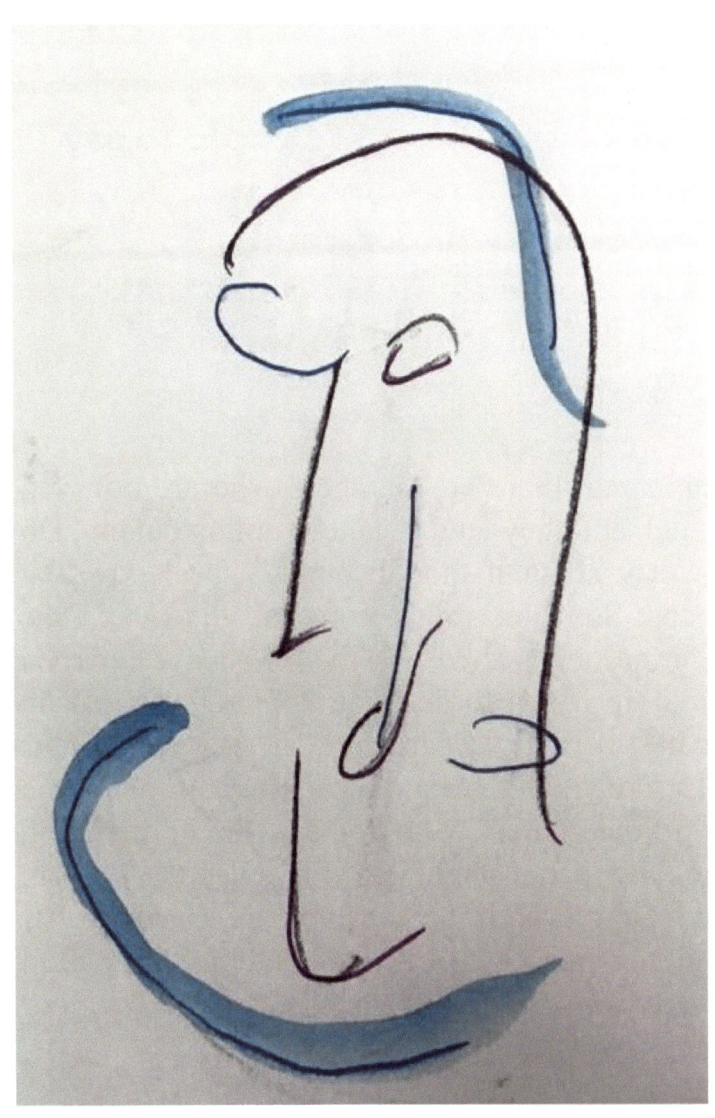

Hope. Transitioned Uncertainties

Retitled Watercolor on paper canvas with sketch tones
©2019 Dr. Peirsol

26. Insecurities cause people to say and do things they do not necessarily understand. Unresolved emotions can make people pounce at a moment's notice.

Be prepared, there are Campers who are not well adjusted, and they tend to take it out on others. Do not worry about it though but just be ready if it happens. Someone might come at you out of the blue in an unexpected possibly twisted way when all you are trying to do is be yourself and just do your best. These experiences, if they come your way, make you appreciate what you have and to be grateful that you are who you are. So, in effect, no matter how bad it might get, if this happens to you, learn from it even if it means you are learning what you do not want to do. This tip is definitely a good one to keep in mind so you can be sure to keep your bearings when stuff starts flying.

27. Get to know your roommate and hope to God they are funny.

If you have to bunk up with someone then this is a critical tip. This jewel of a person is either a comic relief or a dreaded headache (or somewhere in between). Nonetheless, it is someone you have to deal with so you might as well make the most of it. Ultimately, they can be someone that is a sounding board or totally unavailable at all. The key is that you make sure you feel safe. You get that, then you are good. Why? Well, your bedroom is your safe haven away from home. Let's hope though, in addition to feeling safe, you have a funny character as a roommate. This is far better than a stick in the mud. This roommate might not become a long-lost friend, but they can be a much-needed support. Regardless, they will have an impact on your life experience at Camp so be sure to be a good mate to them in return.

28. I hope you packed a new sweat suit that is at least one size larger than you normally wear. For some reason, you can get really bloated at Camp.

I guess when your emotions go haywire, your body does too. Bottom line just be prepared if your body changes here and there while your mind and emotions come hither and yond. Do not worry though, somehow, someway your body acclimates more and more as the days go by.

29. Just being comfortable in your own skin can be tough enough sometimes regardless of the circumstances. So, be sure to have some skin lotion at Camp.

Not kidding on this one. You will occasionally feel all dried up emotionally anyway somedays. And, as silly as this tip sounds, especially if you are a guy, trust me, occasionally there might be a point when nothing else but lotion works to sooth you. Remember, every little bit of help goes a long way.

30. Keep in mind, Camp is just practice for life's little games when you get out. So, start hating to lose, and remember, practice was meant to hurt so "gameday" could run smooth.

Sometimes these sport's analogies work. Take it from my nephew, an Olympic gold-medalist, the difference between an Olympian and a great athlete is that the Olympian hates to lose. In other words, loosing is no longer an option. This is the adage or *ethos* each camper should have going into treatment. "Success is my only option!"

Generally speaking, when it comes to training as an athlete, the practice times are usually tougher than game day. What might be remembered most is not necessarily the games that get played but how difficult the practices are to just make it to gameday. Camp is not much different. It can be gut-wrenching day-in and day-out while at Camp as you practice on aspects of your life; but, when you get home, where it is truly a gameday, it will be far easier as long as you have worked hard at Camp now so you will get to coast a little more later on.

31. Keep a daily log, full of reflections morning, noon and night. You will need it years later when you forget how far you have come.

This is a good idea because it will help you realize an important point here or there you may have overlooked earlier in the day. It may take a little extra time, but it will help you put your thoughts together quicker too.

The key here is to realize it will be impossible to take in all the information being tossed around at Camp all the time. So, decide to take an active role in getting all that you can from each day and a daily log can help. In the end, it will also help you later on when it comes time to regroup after Camp; when you can look over your notes in times of needed reflection to reaffirm all the work you have done.

32. In the larger scheme of things, you are actually the lucky one. Contradictory as this may sound, it is probably true most people you know could use a little Camp time themselves.

Lord knows, lots more need a little Camp time that is for sure! This is important because inevitably you will be feeling bad, if not embarrassed, finding yourself "stuck" at Camp; but, it is critical to remember, it is the better person who embraces their shortcomings and willingly makes the effort to change for the better.

In fact, it is not the absence of pathology that defines our mental health but rather our level of awareness of it especially in relation to others in the midst of it all that can make the difference emotionally. Basically, if we are aware of what is going on within and around us then we have a fighting chance to do something about it. Yes, you are indeed the lucky one. You may not agree with this one right away; but, down the road, you will gladly accept this is at least partially true.

33. If you start to feel worse while you are at Camp, then the irony is you are probably getting better. Life is filled with paradoxes and Camp is no exception.

Our feelings, whatever they might be, start to surface because Camp naturally strips away our defenses, leaving us quite vulnerable to whatever raw emotion we may be facing or possibly masking. Whatever it is deep down in there, just let it come on up and out. If not now, then when? If you wait until later and avoid what hurts most, your problems will inevitably get bigger and tougher, sticking around longer and longer, and become much more difficult later on. Better to feel bad now for a short while than to feel bad later for a long while.

34. Pray as if your prayers are already answered even if you do not know how. You need to start feeling as if there are some tangible results out there rather than just hearing about them.

There is enough research to support the notion that prayer can be healing to the body. The activity itself helps. Thus, the crux is it is important to find a Higher Power that works for you. The sooner you do this the better. Do this, not because I said so or others might be telling you to do so, but rather because we all need spiritual direction in some shape or another at some time in our lives. Some Camps provide spiritual guidance, take advantage of it if you can. If not, seek out someone at Camp who appears to be addressing their spiritual needs, preferably a staff member of sorts. Circumstances in life will dictate that we all reach a spiritual crossroad at some point in our life so what better place than Camp. If not now, then when?

35. Reach out to others "like crazy." All pun intended.

We are generally not taught to depend on others; but, when it comes time for Camp, depending upon others in some form or fashion is everything. We find our way not on our own but generally through others. People bearing info we need come as so-called "pointers"; so, be prepared, there will be a lot of pointing going on. So, keep looking to others to help show you the way. And, keep in mind, you do not have to have all the answers before you find the direction you need either. Let others in and they will help you out in the long run.

36. Get used to it, some Campmates will remind you of people in your life- past and present. So, pay attention, it can possibly save you lots of heartache and loads of trouble later.

Unresolved issues are generally the central topic throughout your stay at Camp. More specifically, past experiences get stimulated in the current ones at Camp, with a full range of possibilities, with various people who are similar but certainly not the same as your past. That is a mouth full simply to say certain people are triggers for those old wounds that will resurface in unexpected ways. So, do not be surprised when they do pop up. Just go with the flow and let whatever comes up come out, remembering that it is happening in a safe place with the right people at the right time; and, to not fight it because these certain unresolved things do not just go away. They linger until they are integrated and re-integrated in your psyche; otherwise, they will just keep coming back bigger and bigger, for longer and longer.

37. Load up on food whenever you want. It is not free. Besides, nobody cares at Camp. That is of course if you are not there to learn "how" to eat.

I am not saying gorge yourself. I am simply saying enjoy your meals with the least regard for concern as possible. Dine and savor the bites because it is one of the least arduous pleasures possible at Camp. Hopefully the food is not bad; so, find what you like and have at it. Take in the company you are with too, especially; and, enjoy all the fun and light-heartedness that might come with feasting together. Eating is one of those breaks at Camp that comes with a replenished since of rejuvenation when done. Lord knows, you will need all the rejuvenation you can get. So, do not pass up a "good" meal in and of itself even if the food is certainly not the Ritz.

38. If you are trying to cut back on how much or how little you eat, you will probably be assigned to your own table. It will help. It works better if you pair up though so choose your friends wisely.

This is no laughing matter. Eating is survival so you have to get that right. You will with time so just pace yourself and cherish the moments as opportunities for renewal rather than despair at Camp. This business about choosing your friends wisely is equally as imperative. You will find you have a cluster of acquaintances at Camp and maybe just a select few or just one you seriously share with, if that. Everybody has their stuff to deal with so they might not have enough to go around; but, those that do, try to take it in as best you can and let them give you the support you have been missing just as you try to give them the support they need as well.

39. Early on, when you get feedback from others, which you will, try to "own" what fits whether you feel up to it or not.

When in doubt, it might even be a good idea to say, "That might fit!" until you are doubly sure it does not fit. Otherwise, others might think you are in "denial" already and that is definitely not good. There is a rule or two in some Camps to keep in mind when confronted. You can respond one of many ways but these three in general might hold the key: 1) "thank you, that fits," 2) "that doesn't fit"; or, in some cases, something to the effect 3) "I'll think about that and get back to you."

Otherwise, people get defensive, shut down or just become argumentative, all of which leads to generally not the best results. The idea behind feedback is to help you see your blind spots and to become aware of the unknown or split off parts of you so they can integrate or reintegrate with who you really are. The more connected you are to those dangling parts of you, (the good, the bad and the ugly), the closer you are toward wholeness verses continually perpetuating the otherwise splintered direction in which you may have been headed (e. g., doing the thing or things that got you to Camp in the first place, etc.). So, feedback is good, whether you like it or not; and, it works if you work it by dealing with it properly.

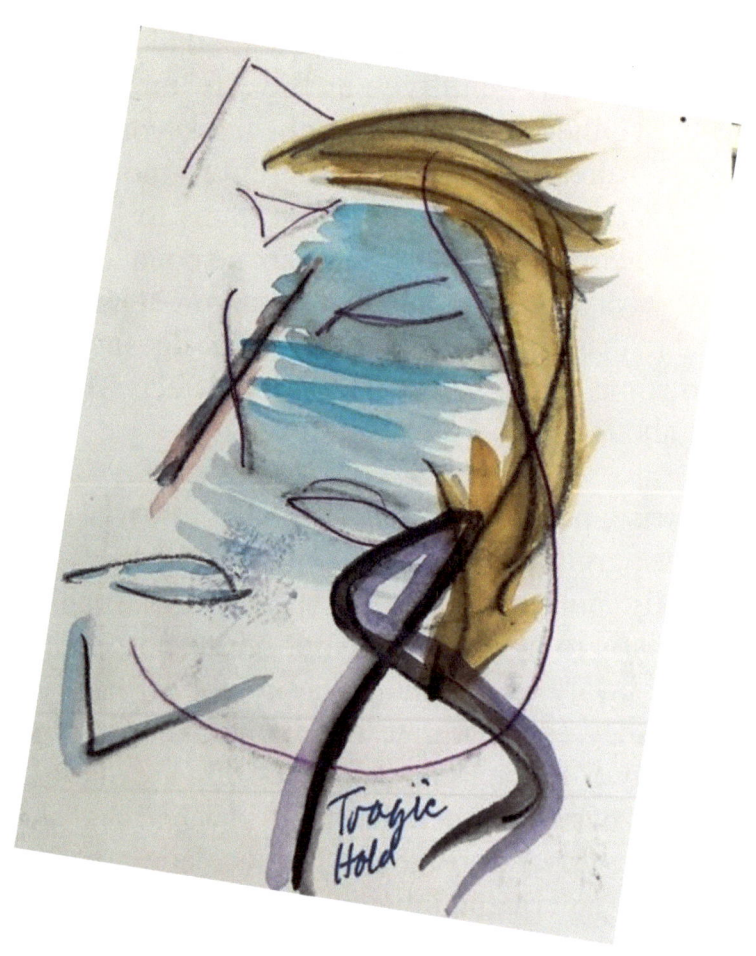

40. Go ahead, let yourself just be a mess at Camp. You are not the exception any more.

This might be hard to swallow at first but start learning to accept the fact you make mistakes and might not have it all together like you had hoped. Everybody has problems, some more than others; and, each of us have certain abilities and certain limitations in responding to our given circumstances. The key here is that you be real about the facts that you face rather than running or masking what truths might otherwise exist. That is it! Nothing radical. Just all on the table without disguise. It is a universal truth we are all flawed in some way as humans; but, it is equally true we all have redeemable qualities worth saving and cherishing, too. It is in blending these blemishes with what is working that makes a broken Camper whole.

41. Get used to having real tough days at Camp. The more quickly you learn to sit in it when you hurt, the more quickly you actually learn to get out of it before you leave.

Camp is a mixed bag. You might have some of the most profound catharsis ever, and experience the most incredible relief possible; and, at the same time, you might reach your deepest, darkest moment ever and have an excruciating heartache that goes sometimes to the depth of the soul. With this tip in mind, try to remember every day is different so you will not always know what is coming, whether or not you will feel good, or what. The truth is however that every day will get better and better at Camp as long as you are working on all that is put in front of you. Remember, all we have to deal with today is today. The therapy and collateral activities are all there for this reason- to make you feel better even if for a while you feel really bad. Hang in there! It does get better.

42. You will soon learn Camp is the "trial and error" test of all tests. So, study hard at Camp while you have to. Most everything in life afterwards by comparison will feel like a breeze.

Whatever comes your way after Camp will not faze you as much as it would have otherwise had you not been to Camp. That is just the way it is. It does not mean that when you get out it will all be easy. It just means the depth to which you go while at Camp prepares you later in life to handle what comes your way more readily. Now, this is only true if you take Camp on with every fiber of your being and put your whole heart and soul into it. So, do not cut corners or gloss over things. Dig deep and explore all your options openly and fully. Soon and very soon, it will be more of a breeze.

43. Do not just think your way through Camp. Remember, your best thinking got you there.

Feelings are deceptive. They are what they are and cannot always be rationalized in the end. So, do not even try to reason your way out of them. Sometimes feelings just need to be felt to be understood just like what you think sometimes needs to be said to be heard. The problem is we just are not well versed while growing up on how to deal with certain feelings when they do surface. And, it is usually our experiences in retrospect that are the teachers for us when it comes to our feelings. Since our feelings usually linger for a while and many times show up after the fact, it sometimes takes retracing the experience to bring what you think and what you feel up to speed. So, while retracing your steps, grant your feelings amnesty the next time they come around. They have earned it just for you.

44. If you think having to go to Camp is bad. Try getting kicked out.

Think about it, you remove yourself from community to pull it together at Camp and then you cannot even put it together while there? Not good. Be prepared, there will be Campers who are just passing through and not ready to get the message they need to hear. Watch them but do not follow them. One Camper, for example, gave the housekeeper a $100 bill to clean up his room for his stay and to get him some instant coffee on the hush. This Camper unfortunately was eventually asked to leave because they inevitably got in trouble here and there or just did not show up for groups like they were supposed to. I have always wondered how this Camper might be doing today because I really liked them. They were really bright and funny too. I can only hope now that they are okay. Do not be this person. Everyone around you at Camp cares in some way about your welfare just by association. When one fails everyone feels it. I would much rather know you made it through treatment than to have not succeeded at all.

In other words, do not get kicked out even if it gets bad for you at Camp. There are Camp counselors and Campers alike that think you matter and have sincere compassion for your well-being. Let them in and let them give you what you might need even if you think or feel they cannot. If after all is said and done, and you still do not feel understood, all you have to do is keep sharing just like in *Finding Nemo* when Dory says, "just keep swimming!"

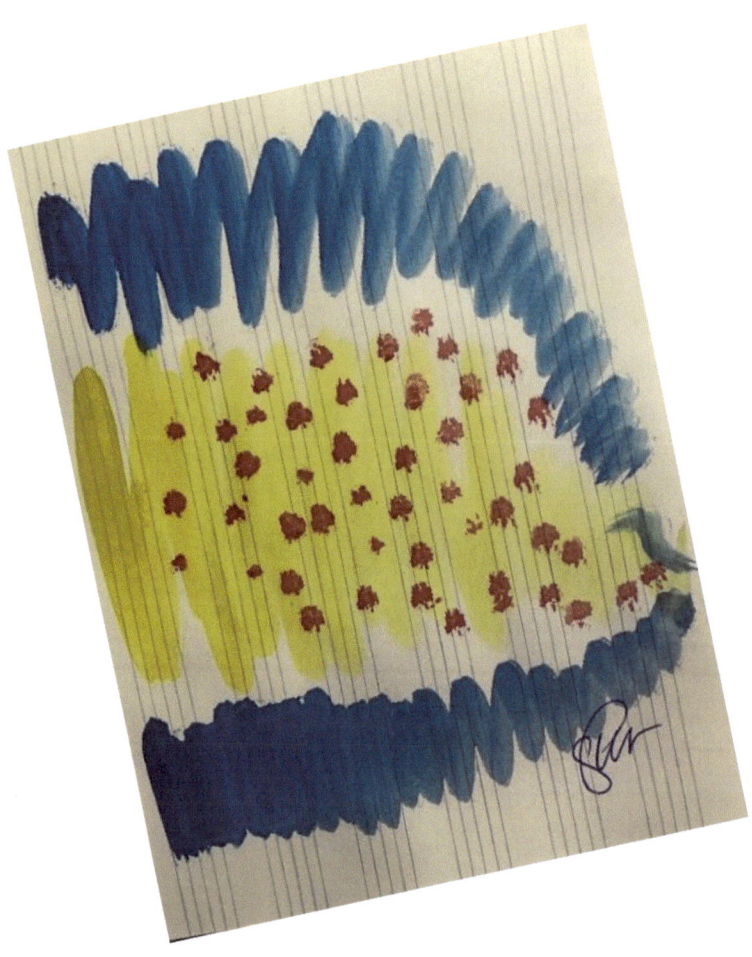

45. Don't pack too heavy. If flying to Camp, save the extra $25 bucks you would spend on that second piece of luggage. You will need the cash for the devotional book you forgot.

Do not forget to bring some extra cash. You might not be able to keep it on your person the whole time; but, you will at least have some extra change for the book store accessories, etc. There are sometimes good books that might help soothe your soul, for example. Find one you like, it could be a nice diversion if anything, and possibly provide the certain insights you need just at the right moment. Besides, moseying around in the gift shop, if there is one, can be a nice distraction.

If there is no gift shop, at least get on-line at some point if you can (with permission of course) and shop on Amazon for a book *The Wisdom of No Escape* by Pema Chodron. Get it shipped. It will help you have a far better perspective about having to be at Camp.

46. At Camp, gravitate to those who are laughing at themselves. They usually "get it" and it will start to rub off on you.

It takes incredible emotional and mental stamina to be able to make fun of oneself in a healthy way. It is an attribute that is sometimes rarely found so when you see it make sure you get as close to it as you can. It reveals that this someone has befriended possibly their demons and has lived long enough to be able to put whatever ails them into perspective to see the humor possibly surround whatever it is. You will be able to tell if it is sincere if they can laugh and equally cry genuinely without skirting the issues. Humor comes as a reward for grasping the big picture. They somehow find a way to approach life with endless openness, curiosity, and confident commitment; and, they somehow seem to be fully assured in the process that whatever comes down the pike will be okay. This is not always the case but if this level of quiet contentment is laughing nearby then do not pass it up.

47. Plan to stay longer at Camp if need be. Otherwise, it could cost you a whole lot more later.

You have made it this far so do not cut yourself short. Go the distance if you need to; miss Thanksgiving Dinner and the holidays if you have to. It is okay. There will be time to celebrate with loved ones later. They will be okay, and they can wait if need be. You, on the other hand, need to be sure you are okay, good to go, and ready when discharge time comes. There is no rush to getting better. Besides, getting better generally has its own timetable.

48. While at Camp, when the time is right, reach out to your family even if you think the time is not right. The more aware of how "out of control" you may have been indicates how much more "in control" you may have ultimately become.

With family and loved ones, this idea gets tested best. Conversations with those closest will always be different from conversations with others. Some might be similar but never the same. When you spend hours on end with Campmates and only 10 or 15 minutes here and there with family or loved ones over the phone, or here and there in visitation for an evening or afternoon, you might find yourself much freer to more fully express what you really think or feel than you ever have before. This is good. Those brief moments with loved ones when you are feeling freer are snapshots into how Camp is coming along. Test the water. See if this sense of wholeness is getting expressed where it matters most (with loved ones) and compare notes along the way with Campmates on how you might be coming along.

49. Every day take time to look at the sky. There **is** life going on outside of Camp somewhere.

When you look at the sun or at the moon while at Camp, remember they are shining on other parts of the world somewhere. A beach somewhere out there is getting loads of sun right now and you can take a break from Camp by imagining yourself being there on whatever imaginary shore that might be. Soon you will be out of Camp and able to explore the world all over again. The beautiful parts of the world have not gone away. They are still out there somewhere waiting for you when you get out.

50. "Healing takes time" is cliché for "I'm stuck, and it sucks!"

Nothing worse than being in a moment you do not like while all the while you are fully aware that the current time must pass before you can either change the circumstance or be beyond the disappointing experience itself. There is no way out. You are there and that is it. The key here is that at Camp we have to be present with ourselves and others regardless of what might be going on. By being present we are alive living life. We may not like it, but it is our life. Our thoughts might go here and there, and our emotions might swing up and down; but, in the end, we are where we are as we are now. It is not tomorrow. It is not yesterday. It is just today. If we can capture this moment, then we are more fully connected to our experience. This is important because those experiences we disconnect with are the very ones that might have brought us to Camp in the first place; so, learn to stay connected even if it sucks knowing full well that whatever it is will somehow someway get absorbed in our masterful psyche at some time. Once it does, it naturally starts to sort itself out as it should when it should. That is how it works. Remember, on those days when the best you can do is just show up, trust your being present is enough.

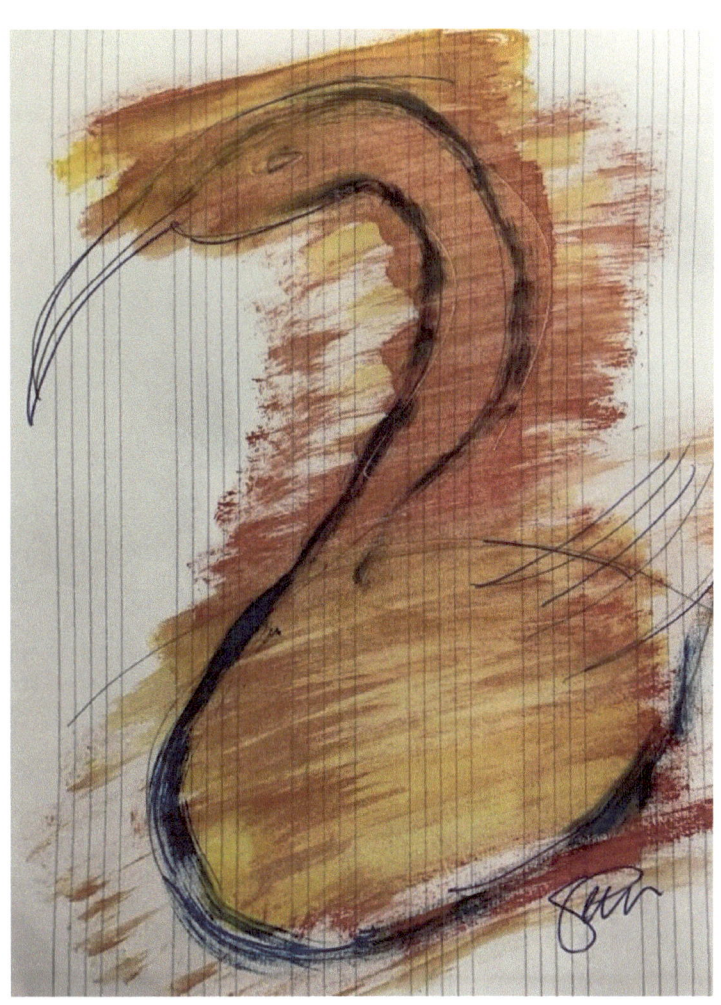

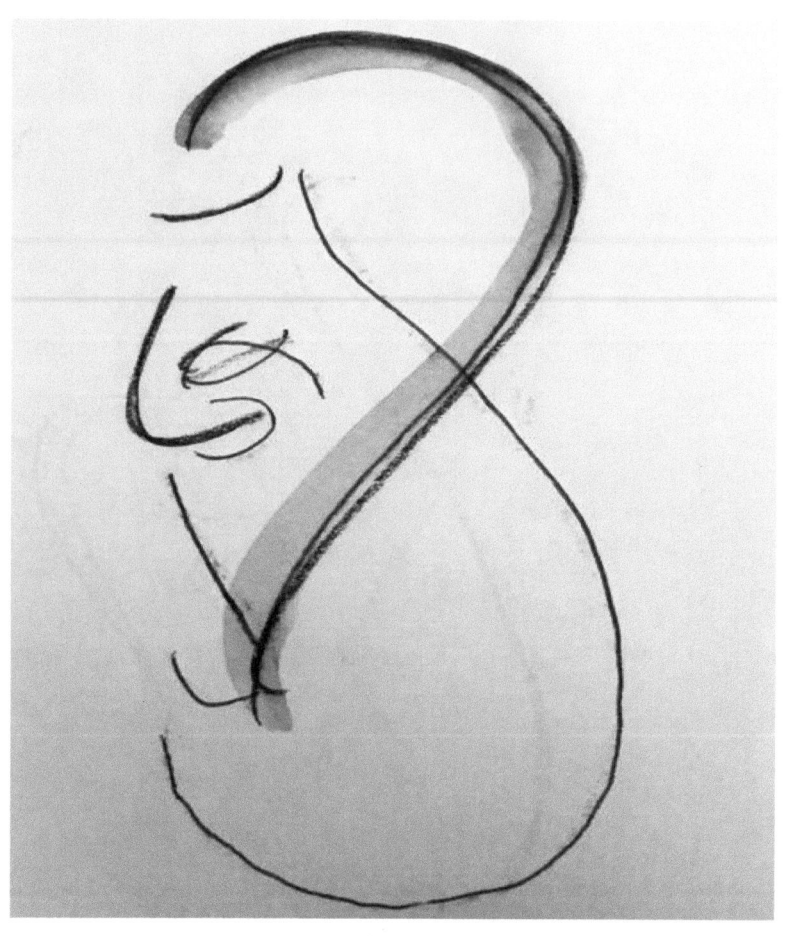

Options. Laughter's Momentary Bliss

Retitled watercolor on paper canvas with sketch tones.
©2019 Dr. Peirsol

51. The 1ˢᵗ Step in a 12-Step program tells us we are powerless over something and this so called "thing" has caused our life to become unmanageable in some way at some juncture. In other words, at some point in our life, we did not quit whatever this "thing" was soon enough while we were ahead.

But here is the catch, if we stop this "thing" just for one day today, then we are already ahead. Here is one-day-at-a-time notion. Sometimes we do not stop what we are doing because we will regret what we may have lost already and have to face that which is so drastically missing. We somehow hang onto thinking that whatever we are doing that is seemingly not working very well will somehow bring itself forward, making it all better in our own imaginary way; that there is still time and not defeat is in site, yet. But, all the while, you have been kicked in the teeth and pushed to the curb.

The key here is in reversing the cycle just by some degree in the opposite direction. It does not even have to be a complete turnaround to get this. Instead of chasing your own tail, just turn around a little bit and you are already on your way. Catch this tip and you are off to a great start.

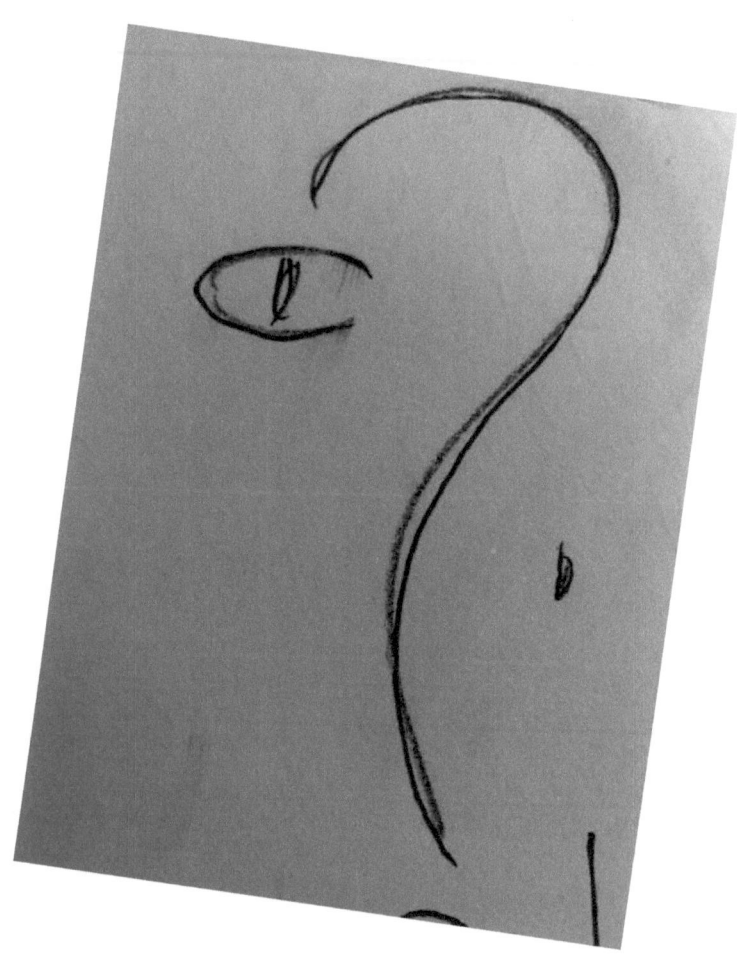

52. Make Camp your home for now. Besides, if you were really comfortable in your own home, you probably would not be at Camp in the first place.

It is easier to hang onto what you feel you might be missing while at Camp than it is sometimes to let the past go. The idea though is to let go so you can find relief from the thing that got you there in first place. That is why it is important to make Camp your home while you can. It is a place for rebirth and renewal that sometimes takes starting anew from a whole different place. When you really think about it, it could be a lot worse. Just imagine having the problems you feel you are facing and nowhere else to go? At least there is Camp.

53. Get to know those so called "experiential" therapists as best you can. They are generally a lot more fun and definitely the "go to" people when the going gets tough.

These experiential therapists, if you have them at your Campsite, are not all entangled in the quagmire of the counseling arena most times. They get to come in the back door by wringing out the proverbial sponge of your emotions to clear the way for you to process more and more as the weeks move along at Camp. By doing certain therapeutic activities, typically physical or artistic in nature, they find a way to help you get Camp off your mind. Where this comes in handy is if your sponge gets too water-logged let's say because your therapist for example is not getting you. You can go to them if after talking to your therapist does not work. You can see one of them to brainstorm certain options. One Camper, for example, had their therapist taking their anger out on them by not reinforcing their progress. As a result, the patient was feeling suppressed and shunned in therapy, put to the side and not attended to. Well, the Camper talked to the experiential staff; and *voila* another therapist showed up one day in group for the Camper unexpectedly, specifically to ensure that the

Camper felt reinforced and acknowledged. That is called being connected.

Remember, find that objective outsider at Camp if you can, even if there is not this experiential therapy going on. In other words, there is always someone around who can see whatever it is that is bothering you from a better angle.

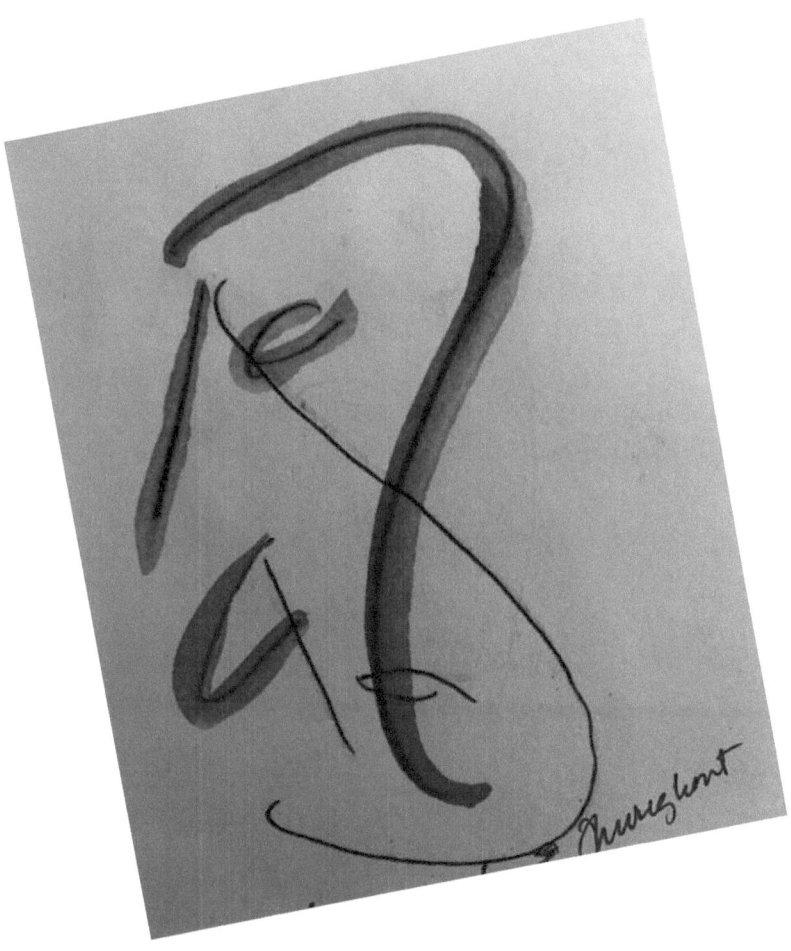

54. "Setting boundaries" could be a nice southern way of telling people off so no one gets hurt. Remember, Camp by in large is a sophisticated crash course in learning how to win or lose gracefully without hurting yourself or someone else in the process.

This one is interesting because it is what otherwise could be considered the political correctness of Camp. Instead of doing what you are doing the way you are doing it, Camp offers you try the same thing but, in another way, to see if it works better. Here is the catch, all this comes with a certain spoken and unspoken language only Camp can teach. After you are there a while you will know what I mean. Many times, we are looking for the right thing but just going about it the wrong way. Camp gives you the opportunity of coming in the back door to a problem in a more effective way. After a while, you will realize that all along you may have been trying to get at the same thing that Camp teaches you to do eventually, just differently. All you needed was a little tweak here or there to get there.

55. At some Campsites, not having any real coffee sucks. Hang in there. You might get lucky and eventually meet someone who has a stash.

There are rules at Camp we may not fully agree with, including no coffee if that is the case at your Campsite. But, upon admission many Campers are just so ready for a change they will agree to anything just to get on with it. Once the dust settles though, it all starts to creep in on you and you might wonder what in the world you have gotten yourself into. Trust me, there will be pleasant surprises that contradict or challenge the rules so rather than fight it I am encouraging you to just go with it. Before long, the rules tend to bend anyway here and there just by the very nature of Camp itself. As long as you are not violating yourself or others in the process, learning to live within Camp's limits is by itself a therapeutic exercise. Besides, when you get out, it makes you appreciate all the comforts of home even more. Hint: *Sanka* is not all that bad by the way.

56. Be prepared for someone at Camp to not like you. Do not sweat it though because you have always needed tougher skin anyway.

This one can be painful. Why? Well, most Campers are very sensitive for starters. Second, it will probably come out of nowhere, so first and foremost do not feel like you should have seen it coming except maybe for this tip here. Third, it will sting and most likely have nothing to do with you for the most part; but, it will have a hidden meaning that will be helpful to you in the end. The work will be to certainly hear what the person has to say but more importantly to try to respond more from within rather than externally as so many times is the case. The situation itself will be different from anything you might have ever experienced but similar in feeling to what you might have felt before in the past. It will be about feelings that get stirred up you will want to address by putting words to the feelings rather than needing necessarily to settle any dispute that may arise. In the end, you might not get to the point where you thank the person for what they said or did; but, you will remember the event(s) itself and the driving force from which your feelings came up, all of which hopefully gets expressed in a new and better way. All-in-all though, however bad it might feel at the time, it will most likely be a catharsis for the other Camper if handled properly by staff and a growth experience for you if processed openly in turn.

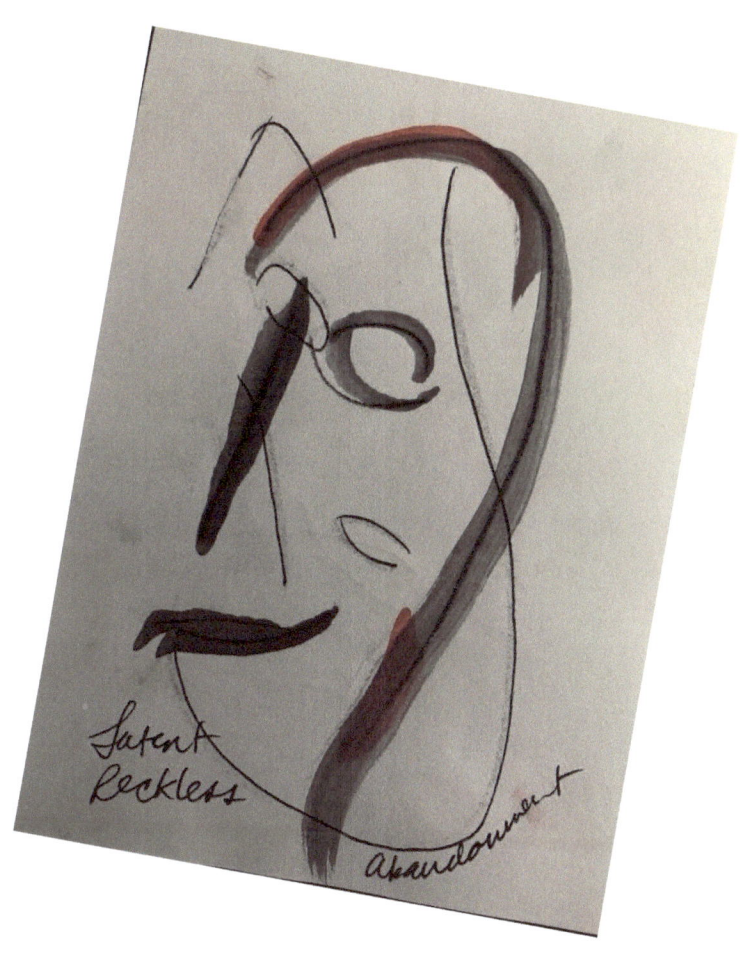

57. The tendency is to feel you should be further along than you are. Remember not to rush things at Camp. You are right where you need to be right now.

Others will seem to be further along than you when in actuality they are just on a different path. You are right where you are and that is good enough for starters. Whatever needs to come will come in its due time as long as you are working at it and remaining open to the process. Again, what you need will come exactly when it should. This Camp thing has a life of its own so let it take shape. It does take time and sometimes that means allowing things to happen on "Camp-Time."

58. Remember, you could use all the feedback you can get, both positively and constructively. There is a limit to everything though, so it is okay to say you have had enough every once and in a while.

There will be more information than you can possibly process while at Camp. It will soon become some kind of blur as the days pass. Do not let that get you overwhelmed. Sensory overload will set in and simply need to be managed by letting that which sinks in to sink in and that which can be let go to be gone. That does not mean don't work at it as hard as you can to get all that you can. It just means do not overdo it to the point you get all worked up.

It is not much different than jumping in and out of a pool. When you get out, you might still be wet, but you are definitely not still in the water treading water. Jump out of the day at Camp just like you might jump out of a pool, so you don't get waterlogged or overcome. For example, go exercise every once and in a while. Do something else other than therapeutic activities. Take a walk. Play a game. Relax. You might still be wet from all of Camp's daily therapeutic activities; but you certainly won't be swimming in over your head when you do take a "time out."

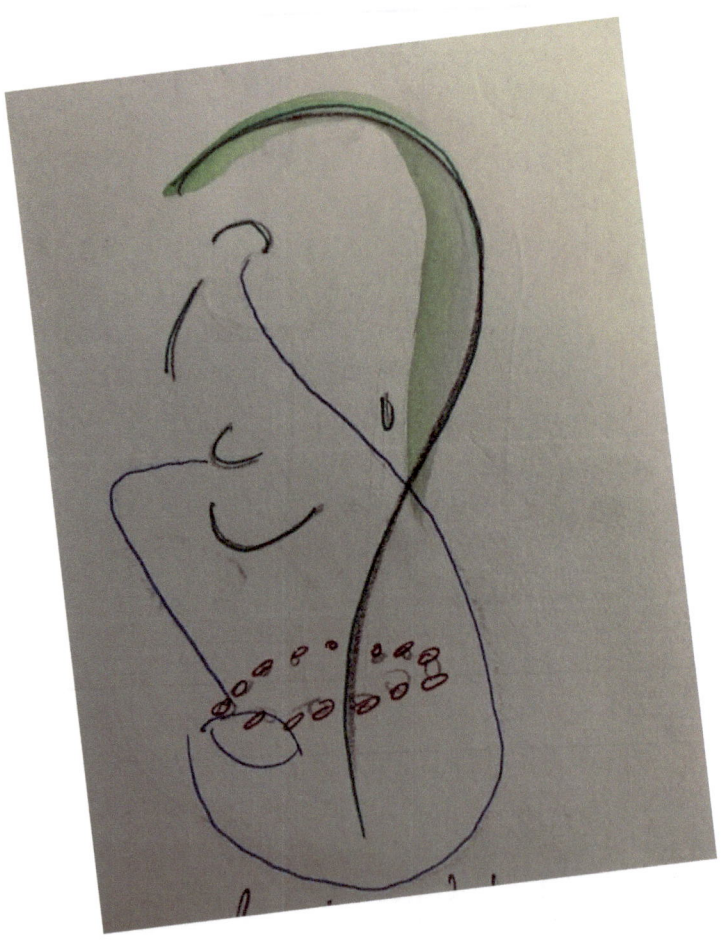

59. When people rub us the wrong way, we sometimes "project" what we are feeling onto them. In other words, we sometimes dodge things about ourselves we really should paying attention to.

Be prepared there will be plenty of Campers that might rub you the wrong way. When this happens, it is important to know and remember that we all mismanage our own feelings here or there in our life. The greater import here however is knowing when you mismanage your feelings verses just knowing whether or not you do. Since Camp will not always be about getting rid of your problems, but instead more about embracing them, it is equally as important to know what you are doing with your feelings when they arise verses just knowing what feelings they might be. In reality, all you are really trying to do is simply better manage them verses trying to get rid of them. You do this, and far less people will rub you the wrong way anymore.

60. We are all riddled with moods at times, but some are rattled by them more than others. If that is you, do us all a favor and take your meds!

Talk about a safe place to try something new; well, Camp is the place! If you are toying with whether or not to take some meds, just be prudent in knowing that sometimes good medication can make all the difference. And remember, not all meds are taken indefinitely. Many can be a good temporary fix. I always say it is like getting a shot in the arm to help you simply get over the hump. They are not much different than vitamins; you pop one and you just feel better. So, before you kick meds to the curb, keep in mind that meds might be what you are looking for. You will not know until you try them. Remember, many before you have tried them and many more have succeeded with them.

61. Do not forget you will probably be liked more for sharing all you did others probably hated you for; and, before long, you will be smarter for all you did that seemed so stupid.

At the beginning, your story may be overwhelming depending upon whatever led you to Camp. Most stories at Camp though are not pretty regardless. The message here is that there is hope regardless the drama you may be facing. This hope will come more quickly the sooner you tell your story, regardless of how bad it may seem to you right now. The more you tell your story, the more your experience of the story changes. Then, all of the a sudden, you are filled with new ideas, new opportunities, new plans, new images, and ultimately a new outlook because every story takes on a new form the more often it gets shared and exchanged with others.

62. Thinking of those you have hurt certainly hurts. Be open to the idea sometimes what we need most comes from feeling stuck.

We can discover that what comes our way in life provides the very information we basically need for our life to unfold as it should. We might not like it as it is and it certainly might not make our day, but in the end as we continue our journey, we can derive meaningful wisdom from it whether we come to fully understand its meaning, purpose and intent or not. Therein lies the difference between just surviving Camp and whether or not we can thrive at Camp!

62. "You are only human!" can be cliché for "There's no quick fix for regrets!"

The extent of our baggage, and how well we manage these imperfections in life, can be determined by how well we live and cope with our failures. The challenge however is in whether or not we learn from our defeats, whatever they may be; and, more importantly, whether or not we can change in such a way that we are better off as a person for having had the setback(s) in the first place. This is a big part of the work at Camp. Once this process of being able to readily sift through our limits gets engaged however, the rest starts to follow. This process can seem relentless though at times, especially at the beginning. Camp is simply a great starting point. It is in making the most out of whatever shortcomings you have, gathering up all the fragments that remain, with all the resources available to you; and, with all the help of others around you, to be able to sustain you moving forward. Let Camp help you shape your future with this less than perfect but better than not perspective in mind.

63. One quick fix is to start talking about what emotions "you think" you feel even if for now you cannot feel them just yet. Do this and it might be a good indicator Camp is working.

There are so many emotions to deal with it can literally be mind-boggling at times. There are so many in fact some Camps narrow them down to five major ones: anger, loneliness, happiness, sadness, and scared or afraid. Feelings can be so important some groups at Camp have you identify one of the five (or more) you are feeling at the time before you speak just to get the group started. This is because when it comes to mental health, what we say and feel needs to coincide with whatever we may be experiencing. Why? Well, feeling one thing and saying or doing other amounts to "a disconnect" from the self and that is not a good sign. We are looking for congruity and authenticity when it comes to emotions and behavior. This equates to psychologically doing better at a very elementary level; and, as far as Camp is concerned, elementary is very good.

64. "Fulfilled living" and "insanity" sometimes come disguised as the same package. That is why they both come with such a high price!

Living a fulfilled life comes with some dues to pay. Camp is not any different when it comes to managing bouts of insanity. How we acquire fulfilled living and how we address our gradients of insanity will all change as a result of Camp. We cannot keep doing something and expect different results if we want to be fulfilled or expect sanity in our lives.

Displaced fulfilled living is because of our lapses of sanity and vice versa. Eventually, when we finally find what works, we usually discover either because of what did not work. In fact, how fulfilled we become equates to how in touch we might be with how out of touch we might have been. So, welcome whatever insanity you may feel. It is an integral attribute toward being fulfilled. After a while, insanity tends to become a pardoned friend who is no longer a menacing foe, and will in all actuality help keep you on the road to fulfillment.

65. You will discover "insanity" can be innovation in a pinch. At Camp, you will quickly discover just how smart it can be, especially once you realize you are not that crazy after all.

Insanity as a loosely used term, taken at face value, can be really scary because we usually equate it to being "crazy" or "out of touch" with reality. Our initial notion of psychiatric problems really should not be thrown around too loosely though because some 94% of Americans at some point in their life will have a diagnosable mental illness. That pretty much levels the playing field and sets the record straight for some. For the most part though, we can all be questionable at some point. At Camp though, you will soon realize there are gradients of insanity and that the term itself will take on more user friendly, familiar qualities. You will discover we all have phases of it, and when we face it head on it is not as intimidating as you once thought it might be. The problem though is some of us do not know this. The truth about insanity is we all have the opportunity of letting it work for us rather than against us. If we follow what ails us to where it may lead, it will ring true that there really is a hairline fracture between genius and insanity at some point.

Each of us has their own unique genius and it is just in how we are channeling who we are as we are with what we want that sometimes can get the best of us. At Camp, you will hopefully realize and become more comfortable knowing that you have probably been bouncing back and forth between genius and insanity without even knowing it for some time now. Insanity, in other words, may not be such a stranger after all but rather simply a part of the you that just needed a little direction.

66. "Unmanageability" and "Higher Power" go hand-in-hand. After a while, the more of one generally means less of the other.

Everybody experiences unmanageability at some point in their life. The question is whether or not you want to make it a lifestyle. There are things we can do and things we should not do that contribute to whether or not we want the unmanageable life. Some of it happens to us outside of our control or we simply bring it on ourselves for reasons Camp helps to unfold. The core issue though is that we cannot fix this unmanageable tendency all by ourselves. We need strength other than our own until this empowering other, whatever it might be for you, becomes a part of who we are. So, I suggest you not poo-poo the notion of a Higher Power just yet. You might want to give it a fair shake before you do. Who knows you might like it? For many, it sure beats being unmanageable all by your lonesome.

67. The fuse for explosions in life generally stem from unfortunate, unintended and or uncalculated risks, conscious or otherwise. Do not worry, Camp has ample detonators.

Let yourself implode at Camp. It is better to bust-out rather than rust-out. All the activities and interactions organized, planned, and conducted at Camp are intended to give you just enough rope so you do not hurt yourself when you do fall apart if you have not already. It is the right place for everything that has gone so wrong. The sooner you allow for whatever is busted to fall apart, the quicker everybody together can help you put it back together.

68. "Psychosis" might simply suggest we are not able to roll the tape back far enough to maintain our bearings. At Camp, there are plenty of cameras rolling, and tons of film to burn.

If you have been seeing or hearing things that are not there, then be sure you are close to the charge nurse managing your meds. Stick to the meds and they will make all the difference. For the rest of us, we are usually just the opposite: we do not see or hear things that are there, and that is the problem. The crux is seeing and hearing the right things at the right time that will make all the difference regardless of what side of the coin you are on. In other words, if it is not working out for you just yet, then you simply have not seen or heard all that you need to just yet. So, keep looking and keep asking. What you need to hear or see eventually will come along.

69. "Woe is me! I am lost..." is an apt way of putting it. Walk slowly and pitch your tent wisely because Camp is uncharted territory with a busted compass.

There is no set formula to figure life out at Camp. There are simply differing ways of getting here and getting there from wherever we find ourselves. It first starts though with knowing where you are right now. If you are feeling lost and all out of sorts, then you are lost and all out of sorts and that is okay. You will soon realize you are not alone, and everybody is still trying to figure it out, too. Because we are in this together at Camp, that makes figuring it out less of a burden and not such a big problem.

We need each other just where we are even though how we maneuver through Camp is anybody's guess on any given day. The key is to go, to move, to show up, to be just who you are as you are right now. The more you do that the easier the trip in the long run. That is right. Just be who you are; that itself helps you get to where you need to be.

70. Camp might be the only place where you can succeed because of your failures. So, start learning to go with what feels bad sometimes.

This can be a quicker way of getting at what is good. It helps you find something better out of what otherwise had been so bad. In other words, we have to absorb what we feel sometimes. We cannot just fluff feelings off like they are some passing thought or a fleeting idea. And, the more difficult the feeling the less likely we are to embrace it for what it is. But we can. Besides, it is just a feeling. That is all it is. It is not somebody or something out to get us. It is just a bunch of chemicals in the body interacting that need a place to be released and resettle. That is it.

What we think about the feelings and all that is a different ball game. It is just a feeling that houses all the energy we are going to need to sort it all out. So, begin to trust that feelings are actually there for you to help you and not to hurt you. And, even though what we feel sometimes stumble us up, they actually are the pathway to feeling better.

71. True emotional heartaches do not go away completely when you get out of Camp. Some heartache can linger just like bad body odor: no matter where you position yourself, it still stinks.

This is a reality check. The key here is whatever has thrown your life into a tailspin does not go away completely when you get out. It simply gets redistributed throughout the rest of your life. At Camp, you are simply trying to find a place to put it for now. This is neither good nor bad, it "just is" a sort of thing we have to learn to cope with. Rather than stay stuck in regret or full of remorse over the past, for example, Camp is a place where new skills and techniques can help you find rest from what is so wearisome. It provides the means to a better future and a new hope for a life to look forward to again. In other words, do not stay stuck downwind at Camp but rather find that proverbial updraft in all that you do there. A disguised refreshing fragrance is waiting to help you feel restored again.

72. At Camp, I suggest you not refuse to try new meds. Who knows, you might feel better.

This will not apply to everybody but to those it does pay attention. Regular advances are being made with the way they make psychotropic medication these days. It works and might be the ticket to a new lease on life if you give it a shot. So, don't shy away from it or get lost in feeling like there is something wrong with you if you need to take meds. It is no different taking medication for your mental health than it is taking meds for most any other reason. Plain and simple, they are there to heal and help you feel better again. Shoot, if only life were always that simple. "You mean all I have to do is take a pill and *voila* that will help me feel better again? Geez and heck fire, sign me up!"

73. Since Camp is a "get it together" campaign, how you account for what has "gone wrong" will be one of those nagging questions even when you get out.

The true test will be whether or not this questioning voice is becoming a gentler, fainter whisper by the time you get out. You will have a lifetime to ponder the "why" of your circumstances; but, for now, while you are at Camp, the question needs to become "How?" How do I adjust to the cards that have been dealt me? How can I make a change for the better with this or that? How do I handle this feeling or that one? How can I take what I am learning and apply it to my circumstances?

The "How To" questions could become just as endless, but they have more tangible results. Now, do not get me wrong, addressing "why" is important but it is not the end all because its answer could be a long-time coming and remain endlessly without closure. So, the more you can discover "how to" respond to your situation then the less likely you will question "why" you are in your predicament.

74. When it hurts most at Camp, we realize "loving our neighbor as we love ourselves" actually means we can no longer gather up the fragments that remain without "others loving us more than we love ourselves."

Reaching the end of your tether and living to talk about it is also a fete unto itself. It is definitely to be applauded and to never be taken lightly in the process. While hanging on for dear life though at the end of the rope, we can only resurface with renewed life, vim, and vigor if and only if we are connected to those around us while coming through it. Bottom line: you cannot make it without the person next to you at Camp, encouraging you and supporting you along the way. Go ahead, let them in! It will make all the difference.

75. One critical crux of Camp is that it makes you experience compassion. Sometimes feeling bad is a way to realize you matter.

I cannot seem to say it enough but those around you are a key component to how well your experience at Camp will go, much less in life. From the cook to the janitor, they all have an impact on your outcome. The good news is you can be as miserable as you might feel, and it will not matter. Those at Camp will still be there for you in the morning. That is how it works. Talk about team work? Camp might be the best consummate makeshift team you will ever experience. So, do not forget what you have to offer, regardless of how bad it might be; it will be equally as priceless for your Campmates as their being there for you will be.

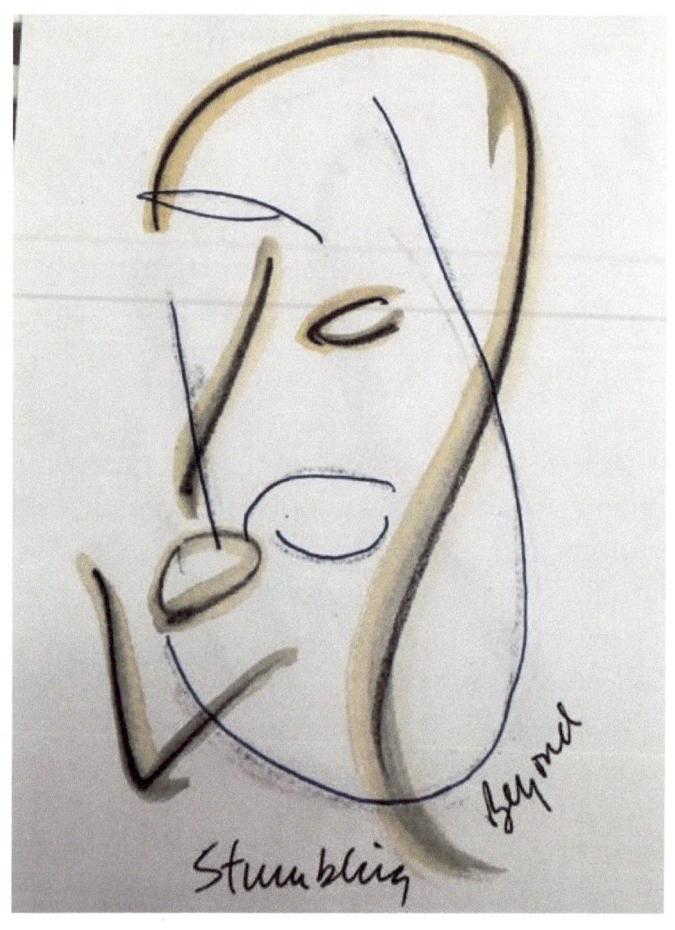

Beyond. Renewed Vigor

Retitled watercolor on paper canvas with sketch tones
©2019 Dr. Peirsol

Many thanks to Becky Benson from Orlando, Florida, and her tireless efforts to edit material for this book. Becky, you are always a cut above, a stellar example of a true friend and confidant.

Much gratitude to my lovely wife, Amy, who put up with my schedule, the multiple hours to write this book, and all the hassles that came with it. Without her, this book would not have been possible.

In addition, this book is dedicated to both my mother and father who in their wisdom were able to provide me with the much needed understanding to be able to help others as a clinical psychotherapist; and, to my brother and sister who over the years have tolerated me and supported me at the same time, loving me for who I am in spite of my shortcomings. In addition, this book is dedicated to *Gary Wakstein* of Panama City Beach, Florida, for his personal sacrifice as a friend, for all his love, support, and extreme patience with me that has made all the difference.

My endless gratitude also to all those who have of late helped me personally and professionally as a person and a clinician. Much gratitude and many thanks to Dr. Joseph DeLuca of Orlando, Florida; Dr. David Parker of Winter Park, Florida; Dr. John Adler of Savannah, Georgia; Dr. A. Banjoko of

Savannah, Georgia and Kim Christiansen & Lisa Oliver of Savannah, Georgia.

This book is Part III of the series *Let's Get Better*. This series includes the following in print or in the process of being published with Amazon Press:

Part I: *Psychotherapy: Let's Get Better*

Part II: *Psychotherapy from the Patient's Perspective: Let's Get Better*
                 forthcoming in the summer, 2019.

Part III (Vol I): *Welcome to Camp I: Let's Get Better*

Part IV (Vol II): *Welcome to Camp II: Let's Get Better*

Part V (Vol III): *Welcome to Camp III: Let's Get Better*

Other writings by Dr. Peirsol include the following and is available by Amazon Press:

Bipolar Depression: Up & Down and All Around